Herbs for Depression and Anxiety

LEARN HOW TO RELIEVE THE SYMPTOMS OF DEPRESSION AND ANXIETY, ANXIETY DISORDER, PANIC ATTACKS AND STRESS MANAGEMENT

By

Dermot Farrell

www.healbodymindandspirit.com

MEDICAL DISCLAIMER

The information in this book is not intended to replace professional medical supervision. Depression and anxiety are potentially serious health conditions and should be regarded with respect. The information in this book is highly effective and it will definitely reduce mental tensions and unhappiness of nearly every person, who earnestly uses the herbs and techniques outlined within. In some cases a cure may take place; however, there is no guarantee that depression and anxiety will be completely cured. Prior to reducing or stopping anti-depressants or anxiolytic medications, do consult with a qualified physician.

Free Gifts

Bonus #1 – Grab Free Books!!!!!!!!

As a way of saying thank you for downloading this book I would like to give you two free books, which are available exclusively for my readers. The free book "Juicing for Health – 35 Juicing Recipes for Everyday Health Problems", is packed full of useful healthy juice recipes and Success Hacks - 31 Mind-Set Hacks to Increase Productivity and Career Success, is packed full of helpful mind hacks for developing a more dynamic and enjoyable lifestyle!

Please go to my blog page and sign up here:

www.healbodymindandspirit.com

You will receive the two free eBooks, plus weekly updates and even free eBooks!

Bonus#2 - Bonus Video Series

You can check out my YouTube channel, which has lots of health related videos

Please copy the following link into your browser, to access an introduction to herbal remedies video. If you then go to my channel and click playlists, you will find lots of videos on herbs for health:

http://y2u.be/VJZ_Kc_dpL4

If you find it too awkward to type in this code, then you can also find my channel by typing in **www.healbodymindandspirit.com** into the YouTube search bar!

Table of Contents`

Chapter One - Herbs and Mental Health

Note: This chapter is quite long and a little technical, so if you just want to check out the herbs, then skip ahead to chapter two. However, since the aim of this book is to provide the reader with herbal remedies, which can either supplement or in some cases completely replace allopathic medication, it makes sense to take at least a quick read through this chapter, prior to adding in herbs or substituting herbs for allopathic medications. After all it is your mental-emotional health, which we are talking about. So please do take at least a quick look through this chapter and proceed carefully, this way you can gain a benefit from herbs with little or no downsides.

The use of herbal treatments for anxiety, depression and neurotic symptoms has been on the increase over the last few years. The reason for this increase, in herbal usage, probably boils down to the near epidemic levels of anxiety and depression, in society today.

Here are some interesting mental health statistics from the USA:

- 3.1% of Americans suffer from General Anxiety Disorder (GAD).

- 2.7% of Americans suffer from Panic Disorder.

- 6.8% of Americans suffer from Social Anxiety Disorder.

- 1% suffers from Obsessive Compulsive Disorder (OCD).

- 6.7% of Americans suffer from depression.

That's an enormous percentage of the US population, who suffer from depression, anxiety and other mild forms of mental ill health. Even if we look away from America and compare with the World health Organisation (WHO), and their findings, regarding global levels of depression, wherein they found that 350 million people worldwide suffer from depression. Taking in a global population of approximately 7.125 billion; 350 million represents approximately 5% of the world population. So America is not alone in having such a big problem with anxiety, depression and various neurotic disorders.

So what can we do about it?

Well one option is to take medication. Medication has received a bad rap lately, with an emphasize on the strong side effects, which go with them, and how they basically act as a crutch rather than a cure.

Actually medication does have its place. The great thing about anti-depressive; anxiolytic and anti- neurotic medication is that it can act as a stop gap, whereby some degree of normality can return, to a person's life, and the downward spiral of mental degeneration can be slowed down and even halted. So as a short-term solution medication is just great. The reason why medication doesn't work out well, in the long-term, is because they are all focused on treating symptoms rather than causes. So as a long-term solution medication doesn't work out well at all.

Western pharmaceutical know-how took a quantum leap in the 1960's, and as a consequence of this, a kind of hubris developed, in allopathic medicine, whereby doctors felt that anytime soon a pill would be developed which would cure all forms of ill health. However, there was a flaw in this thinking and the flaw was to see a human being as a walking talking biochemical phenomena. Of course we are biochemical miracles, but we are far more than just a bunch of cool hardware. We also possess very complicated software (the software been our thoughts and our feelings).

We can call this software the 'ghost in the machine', and this overly mechanical based medical model, completely overlooked the role of thoughts and feelings on our mental health.

9

So yes drugs can act as a stop gap, but in the long-term the only way to cure anxiety, depression and various neuroses is to work on making life changes. Reading good books, attending self-help courses, meeting with mental health professional (counsellors, therapists etc.), making life style changes (changes in diet, exercise, economic decisions about how you are living your life, moving house, city etc.), and basically working through the issues in your life, which are causing you so much mental and emotional upset in the first place.

So when we think about it, it is pretty obvious that we can only improve our emotional lives via long-term efforts to improve our life in general.

Why use Herbs to Treat Anxiety and Depression

So where do herbs come into play?

Herbs are quite effective at treating symptoms of depression and anxiety. In some cases they are as strong in action, as allopathic medications, whilst in other cases they are less effective. In this sense they also act as a stop gap to worsening mental health conditions and as a way to get things back to normal, at least to some degree.

However, herbs also have other significant benefits, which allopathic medications cannot compete with.

1. Herbs Have Far Less Side Effects

Because herbs are naturally occurring, they work in a slower and more moderate manner. This has the disadvantage of making the herb slower to take effect. However, when compared with the molecules of allopathic medications, they are far smaller and result in fewer side effects. While many allopathic medications produce considerable side effects, which can include long-term physical health problems, herbs tend to have very few side effects and most of the side effects tend to be moderate in nature.

2. Herbs Have Health Boosting Effects Which Act as a Holistic Tonic

While allopathic medications force the body into producing calming effects, herbs possess many tonics like effects. On one level this means that the herbs may have a boosting effect on our physical health, which is a nice boon, as well as undergoing their positive mental health stimulating effects. But on another level, their tonic like effects may well help to rebalance our overall wellbeing, which in turn may help to permanently cure our anxiety and depression.

Again looking g at the cure for mental-emotional anguish isn't simply about taking a pill, but rather it's about changing our lives, we can see that our mental problems might not just be about thoughts or emotions. Rather our emotional state and even our physical wellbeing may have an effect, which bring on depressive and or anxiety like symptoms.

What is really great, about herbs, is that they balance our physical, mental and emotional health, which can well be an important element in long term cure!

How to Use Herbs Effectively

Ok herbs have some definite advantages over and above allopathic medications. So we just replace anti-depressants and anxiolytic drugs with herbs instead, simple!

Well it's actually a little more complicated than that. Basically if you are suffering from depression, anxiety or other mental health issues there are two options available to you, which are:

1). Either take allopathic medications or herbs and hope for the best.

2). Use a combination of medications (both allopathic and herbal) while making life changes, and working through life issues over a period of time.

Simply put, even though herbs have many benefits, which go above and beyond allopathic medications, they are still largely a stop gap, unless they part of a proper **mental health treatment plan**.

Now a phrase like mental health treatment plan sounds complicated, but actually it's far more straightforward than you may think. If we want a long-term solution, to our emotional problems, then we have to begin by taking responsibility for our actions and making an effort to make some considerable life changes.

Allopathic medications and herbal tonics represent a medical intervention, a stop gap as it were. Now do not underestimate the value of medical intervention. Whether allopathic or herbal, a medical intervention in the case of mental health issues gives us two benefits:

A).   They stop things from going bad to worse. While they don' fix anything per se, they usually slow down the descent into a worsening mental emotional state, and often they bring the mental emotional state back up to a far better degree. So in this sense they act a lot like antibiotics do, when we have a bad infection. They allow a breathing

13

space, an opportunity to return to normality, which is vital when suffering mentally and emotionally.

B).   Apart from bringing things back to a state of normality, they also in some cases, bring about an actual cure. Often times a negative mental – emotional state ends up in a spiral going from bad to worse. Once these negative feelings and thoughts are checked via medications, this spiral is stopped and often times, if the depressive state is a mild one, things will not just return to a normalish state, rather a complete cure will come about.

So we can see how both allopathic and herbal medications can prevent things from getting worse and can even bring about a cure, in some cases. It's well worth trying some drugs and even herbal preparations, in an effort to bring about a cure. However, don't bank upon a cure from either drugs or herbs. In most cases they will help you, but other factors have also to be considered.

The other factors which have to be considered are:

i). External Life   External life issues refer to things like our economic situation, our domestic life situation, our friends and support network (or lack thereof) which can often result in stress, anxiety and depression. Often by taking some

14

time out, to look at our life and see what is disturbing our peace of mind, and then doing something about it, will produce a positive turn around in our mental-emotional state of being.

ii). Internal Life Issues

Internal life issues refers back to our internal psychic state. How we think and feel about ourselves and the world in which we live in. Do we like ourselves or criticise ourselves. Do we feel the world to be a good or a bad place? Do we lack feelings of inner support and love? Do we love ourselves? Can we receive love? Can we give love?

Often we hear about the lives of rich and famous people, and in some cases people who are extremely successful and talented end up living tragic life's, even though there is no external reason which would explain their state.

This situation of somebody who has everything going for them, and yet they feel down and depressed, is a consequence of internal life issues. Often, in our present day society, we tend to focus upon external success and in so doing so we forget that you can have all the money and success in the world, but if you don't feel happy about yourself, then it becomes impossible to be happy about life in general.

Addressing these two major causes of mental-emotional distress is outside the parameters of this book, as there are many factors which must be considered in such cases. However, what we must bear in mind, if we want to have long-term happiness, is to address our internal and external life issues if we want to either achieve a happy inner state or maintain it, even if we already have it.

So drugs and herbs are great, in their own way, but you have to address your life issues, if you want to arrive at long lasting happiness.

How to Approach Drugs Use and Herb Use

If you are feeling unhappy, begin by addressing your external and internal life issues. If this does not do much to alleviate your mental-emotional issues, then go see your doctor, and be open to trying some medication for a little while.

At the same time try out some herbs. As your mood improves maintain both allopathic and herbal medications. Then try backing off the allopathic medications, but do so carefully. Anti-depressants and other anxiolytic drugs take one to two weeks before they begin working, so have patience when you begin using them. Secondly, when you want to stop taking these medicines, it is necessary to back of off them slowly.

Going cold turkey is a bad idea, as often it results in a rebound in depression and anxiety related symptoms.

Often people like to cut out all anti-depressants, as soon as they feel better. Well this is a bad idea, as often once of off the drugs the symptoms will return. Not only do they often return, but on many occasions when the drugs are reincorporated, they no longer work as efficiently as they did before. What we have to note here, is that many anti-depressive and anxiolytic medications have a strong effect on the neurotransmitters in the brain, such as serotonin. Suddenly going cold turkey can make these levels fluctuate widely and really this should be avoided.

Mental health professionals suggest running anti-depressants for a minimum of three months, and usually opt for at least six months. Now there are varying opinions about this, but the one thing to take away from this, is that you don't go cold turkey!

The allopathic viewpoint is to give the depressed or anxious person a good run of time, without any significant levels of depression or anxiety; the idea been that they will get out of the habit of being depressed or anxious. There is some truth in this, in that people get into either negative or positive mental habits, and that the thoughts and feelings which are now either negative or positive, create feedback which helps to maintain this mental state. So having a period without symptoms, thanks to medicine, can sometimes do the trick and also if a person has been suffering through some external tensions, maybe they have been resolved by then. Anyway, the research carried out, suggests that patients who take anti-depressants and anxiolytic drugs for a period of six months or greater tend to demonstrate a better long-term relief from mental distress symptoms than people who take these medications for a shorter time period.

This is where herbs can help. Start using some herbs and keep them up for at least two weeks, so that they will start working. Do bear in mind that herbs are slower to act than allopathic drugs, so it could take two to three weeks before they work fully. Also most herbs are weaker in effect than allopathic drugs, so it is a good idea to try out two or three herbs and keep using them consistently, as in several times a day.

Then after three or four weeks, slowly reduce the allopathic medication. If say you are on two pills a day, for example, then reduce to two pills on Monday, 1.5 pills on Tuesday, then repeat this for the rest of the week, Then on the following week reduce to 1pill on Monday and no pills on Tuesday, and repeat. Then on week three try out Monday half a pill, Tuesday no pill, and by week four try out Monday half a pill, Tuesday and Wednesday no pill. Finally giving up the allopathic medications altogether by week five.

Now this might sound tedious, but once again I cannot over emphasize the need to slowly come down from anti-depressants/ anxiolytic medications. Also, it must be borne in mind that different people have different reactions to medications and herbs.

A Word of Warning

In some cases it is possible to become entirely free of allopathic medications; however, in other cases this will not be possible. The only way to assess this is to take a cautious approach to replacing allopathic medications with herbal ones. If over a period of weeks everything feels good, then continue to wind down the allopathic drugs, but if some symptoms start kicking in again then stop lowering the dosing of allopathic medications and increase them slightly as needs be.

We must remember that we are working with neurotransmitters here, and while we don't want to stay on drugs for life, we must remember that the first course of action is to maintain a reasonable level of mental- emotional stability, whereby we can continue to hold down our job, or continue our studies and of course maintain healthy functional relationships.

So be cautious, when making changes. Ideally you should transition from allopathic medications to herbal remedies and then eventually give up even the herbal remedies. But realistically speaking, this may not be possible. A good way to go through this process is to maintain a daily journal, with dates and responses. Note down the date when you lowered your drug intake and then track your mood over the next few days. Then a week later, if everything has gone well, drop the medication dosage a little bit and gain keep a track on it.

So if the herbs are working it should be possible, at the very least to reduce the intake of allopathic medications and in some cases they can be dropped altogether. However, unless you keep a record it is too easy to forget when you started to reduce the dose and so everything can get out of hand quite quickly. Usually you can drop medications for a week or two without any symptoms, but then suddenly there will be a negative drop in thinking and feeling, so it is vital to keep a record and up the dosages as needs be.

So it is worth attempting to reduce the dosing of allopathic medications, for a couple of reasons. First of all, it feels good mentally to be free of drugs, and secondly herbs have far fewer side effects and are far less likely to cause deterioration in physical health, which is quite the opposite of long-term allopathic mediation usage.

So by all means try to reduce your drug intake, but do it very slowly and be careful. Maybe you will only reduce your allopathic medicine dosage; well even this is an achievement as it means less pressure on your body, because allopathic medicines are harmful for physical health, in the long-term.

Also, in some case it will be possible to completely stop taking allopathic medications and to rely on herbs instead. Well in this case continue with the herbal remedies for a few months and then start reducing the herbal intake, while taking the same action as you did when reducing allopathic drug intake. Once again you may be able to become complete free of herbs, but if not, at least you will become capable of getting by on less herbal remedies.

And this is a vital point, because whether you are taking allopathic medications or herbal remedies, it makes sense to slowly work towards taking minimum doses, and you will only find this out through careful experimentation. As to the reason, for this minimum dosage? Well this is obvious, the lower the dosage, the lower the side effects, although once again remember to go carefully at this and make sure you are feeling good!

Remember the last thing we want is to go cold turkey, whereby you drop dosages too quickly and then have a rebound of symptoms, whereby you end up feeling worse than ever and the old medications possibly end up becoming ineffective. Instead go slowly and give your brain a chance to rebalance. Also, keep a journal and track everything, this way you can work towards lower dosages and possibly even a complete cessation of drugs, without any nasty side effects or rebound!

Why It's Important to Work on Improving Your Life

So what now, two months in and with a bit of luck you are down to using herbs instead of allopathic medications, so what now?

Well this is really good, but for long-term benefits make some life changes and don't wait for two months before you start making life changes. Rather from day one start assessing your life and making some changes. Usually internal life changes, whereby we learn to like ourselves more and be more philosophical etc., takes a long time. So initially, probably the best way forward is to assess your external life and make some changes. In most cases we are stressed out over one or other things, so take some time out to see where you can de-stress yourself.

Maybe a change of scene for a week or two, or maybe work less hours, or change where you live, or some other fairly minor change which is a cause of stress.

It always surprises me when I speak with people who are suffering, in one way or another, how many times I hear about their twenty hour working day, or their domestic problems or about a person who lives in a violent neighbourhood, for example; how they feel so disempowered, as if they cannot change their circumstances, even a little bit.

What amazes me is how often a minor change could bring about a big change. For example, a reduction in working hours, or possibly moving house, or in the last example moving neighbourhood. Sometimes we become so narrow, in our focus, that small changes like these slip by and we don't realise how we can improve things, by these relatively little changes.

This leads onto another important consideration. Often when we are in a distressed state, we are too close to our problems to really see the wood for the trees, so do consider getting some external help. External help could be something as simple as having a chat with a friend or a relative, attending a support group or going to see a counsellor or therapist. Don't be embarrassed, as many of your neighbours are also suffering with mental-emotional issues.

Just look back at the stats listed above. Approximately 5% of the world population is suffering from some sort of mental distress, that's 1 in 20 people! If you live in a neighbourhood of say 5000 people, which means that at any one time 250 people are facing the same kind of anguish as you! Now they probably don't go around shouting this from the treetops, but mental emotional problems are really common, so don't feel as if you are on your own!

So don't feel alone, and do consider getting some help, as there are many people out there who can and will help you, it just takes willingness on your side, to make some life changes.

So in summary, don't be afraid to take allopathic medications. Most of the horror stories, which you have heard about them relate to either ignorance or abuse.

Too many people have been prescribed anti-depressants and anxiolytic medications for years and years, without any supervision at all, and basically they are now addicted to them plus they have lots of physical health problems, because of the long-term side effects of taking these drugs continuously, this is not good. So here we see a case if ignorance.

The other end is of course abuse, whereby one or more drugs are mixed together, into a concoction, in an effort to feed an addiction. Once again this is not good.

So let's put ignorance and abuse to one side and look at the correct application of these drugs. Drugs for relatively mild mental-emotional issues are designed to be used for a relatively short period of time, of approximately 3 to 6 months. Most doctors will recommend this trial period, and if everything is ok they will suggest slowly coming of off them, around this stage. If conditions start to degenerate again, while reducing the medications, then they will suggest a long-term maintenance dose.

So far so good, **where things start to go wrong is long-term unsupervised usage**. So keep in contact with your doctor and like I said try to integrate herbs from the beginning and gently reduce the dosage. Your doctor may not be too enthusiastic about applying some herbs. If this is the case assure him that you are using them to assist the allopathic medications, because they have a role to play when your doctor suggests coming of off the allopathic medications, as they will help to assist your mental emotional state, as you come of off the allopathic drugs.

What if your doctor doesn't suggest coming of the drugs?

Then consider changing doctor, as any doctor who suggests long – term allopathic treatment, without any possibility of either reducing or changing medications is not serving you well.

Too many doctors rely upon allopathic treatments only, because they have no way of really helping their patients, so with no other likely option available, they simply keep on prescribing the drugs.

We all have options, but your doctor may or may not know this. The worldwide allopathic medical system does not as of yet have a comprehensive and effective strategy for dealing with mental health issues, and the terrible stats confirm this. Allopathic medications, while powerful are only one part of the cure. The long-term cure requires either allopathic or herbal interventions, assessment and changes to external lifestyle issues and assessment and changes been made to internal life issues.

So just because your doctor went to medical school does not make him, or her, an expert in mental health. Now while some doctors are great, just be aware, that as a rule of thumb most doctors are not well prepared to deal with mental health issues and they usually depend too much on drug applications.

So as always apply your common sense.

So let's presume you have a good doctor, who wants you to reduce or even stop medication, if at all possible. When you take herbs, they will assist you and help to relieve symptoms and will also act as a great boost, when you start to reduce the allopathic medications. When you come of off the allopathic medications, continue with the herbs, while working through your life issues.

Over time do try to reduce herbs also. Many of the herbs in this book are easy to take; for example chamomile tea is delicious and easy to take. So it's easy to continue with them, but obviously over time do try to reduce herbal intake, so that a stage arrives when you don't have to rely upon allopathic medications or herbs. We want to get to a stage when we are free of all assistance.

So this is basically the approach to take. I know it sounds complicated, but it's not as complicated as it sounds. If you don't like complications, then simply sign up to taking allopathic medications for life, but I warn you they have long-term side effects!

Curing yourself from mental-emotional issues is time consuming, but it can be done. But to do so requires a realisation, that life is complicated and that we have to continually work through life issues, if we want to maintain long-term happiness!

Finally What to Do If You Cannot Get of off the Drugs?

What to do if no matter how many herbs you take that giving up allopathic medications still produces negative side effects?

Well in an ideal world we should be free of all medications, but this may or may not be possible. While I don't condone unnecessary usage of allopathic drugs, I also do condone the necessary use of them!

The majority of people can come off allopathic mental-emotional drugs, but some people simply can't. But that's ok, certainly drug usage can be reduced and a greater level of control and support can be achieved.

While it would be ideal to possess a full recovery, without any assistance of drugs, herbs or counsellors etc., the simple reality is that some people will have to continue with drugs, but improvement is ways possible.

Looking at the herbs which follow in chapter two, they are very simple, but also they are very effective. Also I hope that the simplicity of most of them will reassure you. These herbs are effective, but do remember what has been said in this chapter; that herbs can either assist allopathic medication or even replace it in some cases. But for long-term benefits, do make long-term life changes and keep on making them, that is the real key to happiness.

Also a Word of Warning

While herbs are great they are also chemical compounds and many of them do possess attributes which could be bad for your health. So do make a point of looking through the contraindications section, which is listed at the end of each herb section. By and large herbs are much safer than allopathic drugs, and also they have far less side effects. But sometimes they do have side effects and the can be detrimental, so check the contraindications and always start on a low dose and increase over a period of a week or two, just in case you have a bad reaction to them, which happens sometimes.

Finally do remember that herbs are slow to work and often they are weaker in their effect than allopathic medications, so usually several herbs have to be combined together, so as to have a similar effect as one allopathic medication. But on a positive note they also have fewer side effects.

So take a look at the list of herbs, in chapter two, and do try them out. Also give them a couple of weeks to work. Combine them with allopathic medications, or try them on their own, but do not dismiss them as they are really effective in their own way.

Chapter Two – Common Herbs for Anxiety and Depression

Kava Kava

Kava kava (Piper methysticum) is a popular medicinal plant, which hails form he south pacific islands. The islanders there have used it as a treatment for a variety of mental health issues, over the centuries, which includes depression, anxiety and insomnia.

Kava kava active ingredients are kavalactones, which have been noted for their beneficial effects upon General Anxiety Disorder (GAD). In one study they noted a significant reduction in depressive symptoms. In particular they noted that 26% of the Kava Kava group, where still in remission at the end of the study, which suggests the good long-term effects of Kava Kava on mental health issues.[1]

Kava Kava Safety?

There has been some speculation on the safety of Kava Kava, after it was banned from most European countries, after a spate of deaths in

2002. However, as of 2014 Kava Kava has been found safe and reintroduced into the European market.

The reason for the re-introduction lies in the nature of the initial evidence from 2002, which purported a tie in between liver health and kava kava. A German court found this evidence to be too circumstantial in nature. Since Kava Kava has been used for centuries by the Pacific islanders, it is very likely that Kava Kava is safe. However, like all herbs there are contraindications, so since Kava Kava appears to be a hepatotoxic in some cases, it makes sense to avoid it if you have liver disease; other than that it appears to be pretty safe, and certainly it is quite an effective anti-depressive and an anxiolytic.

How to Take Kava Kava:

Kava Kava usually comes in powder form, where it is mixed with a beverage in a mixer. Simply mix then filter and then drink.

Two tablespoons equate to approximately 30 grams of Kava Kava extract. Start off with one serving a day and increase after a few days if there are no symptoms. Herbs are very safe, but in some case symptoms do arise, as no one herb is ideal for everybody.

Another thing to note, not only with Kava Kava, but also with every herb is that on a positive side they possess far fewer negative side effects, when compared with pharmaceuticals. However, on the other side they are slower to work. So give it around 1.5 to 2 weeks before expecting any noticeable alleviation of symptoms.

Also depression, anxiety and insomnia often go hand in hand. And one thing which Kava kava is really good at is reducing insomnia. If you suffer from insomnia, then take a serving of Kava kava one hour prior to bedtime, in all likelihood you will see a noticeable improvement in symptoms of insomnia, such as difficulty in getting asleep and waking up frequently due to disturbed sleep.

Kava Kava Tea

Many people take Kava Kava with water, but Kava Kava can be mixed with any of your favourite beverages, such as kava Kava tea.

1.	Blend 3tbsp's of kava kava in with 3 cups of water.

2.	Heat for 5 minutes, while stirring occasionally. Some people prefer boiling the mixture while others prefer to take it warm or even cold. Experiment a little and see what works for you. Also, when boiled some people find the kava kava to be stronger, tending to numb the tongue and also for some, strong sedative like effects are noticed when the mixture is boiled. So see what works for you.

3.   Strain and pour.

Also, Kava Kava can be taken cold and it can even be mixed with 7up or sprite, while other options include mixing it with coconut milk.

Many people hate the taste of kava kava while others love it. Experiment and see what works for you!

Kava Kava Contraindications:

•   Alprazolam (Xanax) causes drowsiness. When combined with kava kava this might result in excessive drowsiness levels.

•   Medications which are changed by the liver (Cytochrome P450 1A2 (CYP1A2), (Cytochrome P450 2D6 (CYP2D6) and (Cytochrome P450 2C19 (CYP2C19) might become less effective when combined with kava kava.

•   Levodopa increases dopamine levels in the brain, whereas kava kava reduces dopamine levels. Consequently, kava kava might reduce the effectiveness of levodopa in some cases.

St John's Wort

St John's Worth (Hypericum perforatum) is one of the most famous plants used to treat a wide variety of symptoms including anxiety and depression. It is found in Europe, Asia and the USA and has been popular for at least two thousand years, so it truly has stood the test of time.

St Johns Wort contains two ingredients which provides its many health boosting effects, hyperforin and hypercin.

Hyperforin helps with spasm reduction in the gastro intestinal tract. 2 Also it has been shown to demonstrate significant anti-depressive properties. 3

While hypercin provides a wide range of benefits, which includes wound healing 4, anti-inflammatory 4, antimicrobial 5, sinusitis 6 and seasonal adjustment disorder (SAD) benefits. 7

So, as we can see St Johns Wort can be considered an overall health tonic, as well as a viable treatment for depression.

How does it treat depression?

As of yet we are not sure why, there is some scientific discussion which suggest that maybe hyperformin and hypercin possesses some serotonin boosting effects; serotonin, being the feel good neurotransmitter in our brains.

Whatever, the case St Johns Wort is certainly effective.

Is St Johns Wort Safe?

There have been some concerns over St Johns Wort possessing heavy metals, which are toxic, but in general it appears to be well tolerated by most people. Do your research on any brand of St Johns Wort, which you are thinking of buying, in order to make sure that the quality of that particular product is good. Simply put the name of the vendor into Google and add in the words complaints at the end. For example, "xyz companies St Johns Worth complaints". It's worth your while checking this out as some suppliers seem to have low quality products. Other than this St Johns Wort is usually very well tolerated, by most people.

How to Take St John's Wort:

St Johns Wort can be taking in capsule form, in liquid form and even as an extract, whereby it can be made into a tea. Atypical dosages are approximate 300mg per day.

Contraindications:

•   It is safe to take St John's Wort, as it has been used by countless generations, over the centuries. However, it has been noted that St John's Wort breaks down some of the active components of pharmaceutical drugs in the liver. Consequently, it is contraindicated to take St John's Wort at the same time of ingesting pharmaceuticals, as it may well reduce the effectiveness of the drug. If you are taking prescription drugs, make a point of taking the St John's Wort either several hours before or several hours after the prescription drugs. A three hour gap should be sufficient.

•   Do not take St John's Wort with selective serotonin reuptake inhibitors (SSRI). SSRI's increase serotonin levels, and when combined with St John's Wort, it can boost serotonin levels too high, resulting in a condition called serotonin syndrome.

- Avoid if using oral contraceptives, anti-consultants, theophylline, digoxin, warfarin, triptans or HIV protease inhibitors.

- Do not take during either pregnancy or when breastfeeding.

- Avoid over exposure to the sun if fair skinned.

Valerian

Valerian just like KavKava and St Johns Wort, has been used for hundreds of years as a potent treatment for insomnia, anxiety depression and even as a muscle relaxant.

Valerian possesses valerenic acid, which possesses many great benefits which includes antioxidant properties, liver protection abilities, it is an anti-insomniac and it helps to treat anxiety. 8

Also Valerian has been noted for its sleep promoting effects. In a study of 16 participants a noticeable improvement was recorded in overall sleep patterns. 9

Needless to say, if you have anxiety and depressive symptoms chances are that you might well have some degree of sleep disturbance as well. Certainly it is worth taking valerian if you find it difficult to sleep or suffer from a disturbed sleep pattern.

How to Use Valerian:

Valerian can come as a tablet or as a dry herb. Daily dosages levels are usually around 400mg to 900mg a day for insomnia and anywhere up to 1200mg a day for anxiety. For insomnia take it one hour prior to bedtime. For anxiety take it three times daily.

Contraindications:

- Do not take while on sleeping medication.

- Do not take if pregnant or breastfeeding.

- Do not use before driving or using heavy machinery.

Passionflower

Passionflower is a great mood enhancer. In a 2002 study of patients suffering from General Anxiety Disorder (GAD), they compared the action of passionflower against a well-known anti-anxiety drug (oxazepam) and noted a similar response in the patients who took passionflower as to those who took oxazepam, with two notable exceptions. 10

Firstly the passionflower was slower to produce a result and secondly it produces far less side effects. Slow to act and few side effects are common aspects of herbs, and it must always be borne in mind that the very fact that herbs produce less side effects is because of their gentler action, which also means a slower response time!

How to Take Passionflower:

Passion flower can be taken either as a tea or as a tincture:

Passionflower Tea

1.   Grind 2 grams of passionflower (per cup) into a fine powder.

2.   Add the ground leaves into a cup of water and bring to the boil.

3.   Leave to simmer for 20 minutes.

4.   Strain and drink.

Passionflower Tincture

1.   In order to make a passionflower tincture the leaves, vines and flower buds are used.

2.   In order to make a tincture, it is necessary to mix the plant material with a liquid which will extract the compounds from the herb; this liquid is known as the menstruum. The ratio necessary with is 2:1. The menstruum can be alcohol; otherwise apple cider vinegar can be used instead. The menstruum also acts as a preserver, so the tincture can be used over a long period of time. Usually vodka, brandy or grain

alcohol are used as the alcohol base, do not use beer! It's necessary to have a fairly high percentage of alcohol, so as to preserve the tincture.

3.   To make up the menstruum, mix in alcohol/apple cider vinegar at the ratio of 3:1. So mix the alcohol and water at 3:1 and the menstruum with the passionflower in a ratio of 2:1.

4.   Chop and ground the flower. Add in about 2 ounces (60grams) of passionflower with 4 ounces of menstruum (about 3 ounces (90grams) of alcohol/vinegar to about 1 ounce (30 grams) of water. Place the mix into a blender and blend.

5.   Pour into a glass container (do not use plastic), leave in a dark cool place.

6.   Shake it daily for a period of 14 days.

7.   Strain through several layers of cheesecloth and squeeze out the essence.

8.   Leave this remaining mix to settle overnight, then pour out the clear liquid at the top (decant).

9.   Store in a dark glass container (a tincture bottle is ideal) in a cool dark place.

When you want to use it simply take out a tincture dropper and use 1 -2 drops anywhere from 3 to 5 times daily.

This tincture should last for a long time thanks to the preserving qualities of alcohol/vinegar.

Contraindications:

Do not take if pregnant or breastfeeding.

Chamomile

Chamomile, good old chamomile always tastes really refreshing, but did you know that it does wonders for depression and anxiety? And that back in the day before anti-depressants came along, that atypical treatment for depression was a prescription of chamomile tea?

Chamomile has been used since the days of the pharaohs back in old Egypt. It is a fantastic tonic, which includes terpenoids (terpenoids possess anti-bacterial, anti-carcinogenic properties, and they also have regenerative and anti-oxidant properties), flavonoids (which possess anti-oxidant and anti-inflammatory properties).

Chamomile produces a wide range of benefits, which includes anti-inflammatory, skin problems, stomach problems, insomnia and of course depression.

In a 1995 study of the structure and action of chamomile the researchers noted that chamomile operates in the same way as benzodiazepine receptor targeted anti-anxiety/anti-depressive drugs. 11

How to Take Chamomile:

The most popular way to take chamomile is as a tea. For good anti-anxiety/anti-depressive benefits take at least 3 to 4 cups a day!

Chamomile Tea

1.   Boil water.

2.   Add on heaped teaspoon of dried chamomile leaves.

3.   Simmer for twenty minutes.

4.   Strain and serve.

Contraindications:

•   Watch for excessive drinking of chamomile tea during pregnancy, otherwise it is generally safe to take.

Green Tea

Green tea is really famous, both for its unique tastes and its host of great health benefits, which include anti stress and anti – anxiety properties.

Green tea contains an amino acid (L-theanine), which helps to lower heart rate and blood pressure. In a study of 18 university students, which were divided up into low anxiety versus high anxiety, that the high anxiety group demonstrated a drop in heart rate and blood pressure levels, combined with enhanced alpha bands electroencephalographic activity (which indicates improved reactions

44

times). Simply put, green tea will both relax and stimulate people (in a healthy way) who suffer from anxiety, at one and the same time. 12

The participants, in this study, achieved these results by imbibing 200mg of L-theanine per day, which is equivalent to five cups of green tea a day. Obviously a lot of tea, but doable, if you like drinking green tea. Also, green tea, when taking in large quantities possesses considerable detoxing effects, and can even aid weight loss.

One thing to note, however, is the quality of green tea varies a lot. So shop around and try out different suppliers and figure out which one works best for you!

Lavender

Lavender is famous for its sweet relaxing smells. Lavender is found in many products including lavender soaps and other bathroom products and of course the lavender oil burner, where drops of lavender oil are burnt in a small water container, which sits atop an oil or wax candle burner.

Interestingly lavender is not only sweet smelling, but also it is highly relaxing. For example, if you suffer from insomnia, then try out a lavender oil burner an hour before sleeping. Lavender is extremely relaxing and will induce sleepiness in a small room.

Also, lavender even helps to reduce feelings of anxiety. In one study, on nursing students in Korea, they noted no significant reduction in depressive feelings; however, they did note a marked reduction in anxiety symptoms, when the students wore a necklace containing lavender essence, over the period of one week. 13

Lavender doesn't appear to be a magic cure for depression, however, many depressive patients also suffer from feelings of anxiety, and so lavender could well be one helpful aid for anyone who suffers feeling of anxiety, along with the depression itself.

Equally significant is the effect of lavender on anxiety, since the majority of people suffer from some degree of anxiety, at least some of the time. In our modern daily lives we are under terrific amounts of mental tension, which come about as a consequence of our busy modern lifestyle. So lavender is a herb which should probably be used by all of us from time to time, for its relaxing and de-stressing properties!

Catnip

Catnip (Nepeta cataria) belongs to the genus nepata of the lamiaceae family, and is a popular plant in southern and eastern Europe, the Middle East, central Asia and China.

Catnip is effective in treating a wide variety of health conditions, including skin problems, arthritis, haemorrhoids, indigestion, colic, cramping and even flatulence. Also catnip is an effective treatment for headaches (including migraines) insomnia and anxiety. 14

How to Take Catnip:

Catnip Tincture

1.	In order to make a tincture, it is necessary to mix the plant material with a liquid which will extract the compounds from the herb; this liquid is known as the menstruum. The ratio necessary with is 2:1. The menstruum can be alcohol; otherwise apple cider vinegar can be used instead. The menstruum also acts as a preserver, so the tincture can be used over a long period of time. Usually vodka, brandy or grain alcohol are used as the alcohol base, do not use beer! It's necessary to have a fairly high percentage of alcohol, so as to preserve the tincture.

2.   To make up the menstruum, mix in alcohol/apple cider vinegar at the ratio of 3:1. So mix the alcohol and water at 3:1 and the menstruum with the passionflower in a ratio of 2:1.

3.   Chop and ground the plant. Add in about 2 ounces (60grams) of catnip with 4 ounces of menstruum (about 3 ounces (90grams) of alcohol/vinegar to about 1 ounce (30 grams) of water. Place the mix into a blender and blend.

4.   Pour into a glass container (do not use plastic), leave in a dark cool place.

5.   Shake it daily for a period of 14 days.

6.   Strain through several layers of cheesecloth and squeeze out the essence.

7.   Leave this remaining mix to settle overnight, then pour out the clear liquid at the top (decant).

8.   Store in a dark glass container (a tincture bottle is ideal) in a cool dark place.

Dose: Catnip is usually taking as a tincture or as a tea. In tincture form, take 30 to 90 drops in a 2-4 millilitre tincture

Catnip Tea

1.   Boil water.

2.   Add on heaped teaspoon of dried catnip extract.

3.   Simmer for twenty minutes.

4.   Strain and serve.

Catnip Contraindications:

•   Belonging to the lamiaceae family, it can produce an allergic effect in some cases.

•   Do not take if breastfeeding or pregnant.

•   Catnip can have an effect on the central nervous system. If taken in large doses there may some toxicity, so take a reasonable amount but do not overdo it.

•   Catnip contains verbascoside, which may affect the immune system. Be careful if taking catnip while on immune boosting medication, as there may be a negative interaction.

- Catnip helps to promote sleepiness, but this is contraindicated if you are going to drive a car or bike or work with heavy machinery.

Fennel

Fennel is an extremely healthy herb and a popular one in the diets of a great many people. Benefits of fennel include indigestion, constipation, colic, diarrhoea and flatulence assistance. Also it aids anaemia, respiratory and eye function, blood pressure, heart health and it boosts oestrogen production, which is beneficial for menopausal women.

Fennel is also really helpful with symptoms of anxiety. While there is no good scientific research to back the claim that fennel helps relieve anxiety, there is a lot of anecdotal evidence which suggests that it has a soothing quality.

How to Take Fennel:

For symptoms of anxiety fennel can be taken as aromatherapy oil, either via an oil burner or as drops of fennel oil poured onto a handkerchief.

Been a herb, relaxing benefits take a while to kick in, but often do so within an hour or so. Fennel oil, on a handkerchief, for example, is an excellent way for someone to maintain a soothing effect throughout the day, by simply sniffing the handkerchief whenever they feel anxiety symptoms.

Fennel can also be taken as a tea. As a tea it is a general tonic and is generally considered as soothing and good for health. From an anxiety point of view it will probably produce a better result in oil form, but it's worth trying it out as a tea and seeing how well it works, if nothing else it will certainly have a relaxing and healing effect on the body.

Fennel Contraindications:

• Fennel promotes oestrogen production so should be avoided by anyone who is taking birth control pills, as it may result in a decrease in effectiveness of the north control pills

• Do not take alongside the antibiotic ciprofloxacin as fennel may reduce its absorbency rates.

• Do not take along with Tamoxifen (Nolvadex) as the fennel may interact with the tamoxifen thus resulting in a lessening of its effectiveness.

• Do not take in excessive amount if you are a male, because it can result in excessive oestrogen levels which will have a negative effect on body fat and water levels in the male body, plus possibly a reduction in sex drive.

Ashwagandha

Ashwagandha is an ancient Indian herb, commonly known as the "scripture of longevity", and commonly used in aryuvedic medicine for treating a wide range of conditions, which includes Parkinson's disease, cerebellar ataxia, ADHD, arthritis, high cholesterol levels and diabetes along with a wide range of other health conditions.

Ashwagandha has also been widely used for the treatment of anxiety, although at this stage scientific evidence is only tentative. 15

How to Take Ashwagandha:

Ashwagandha can be taken as a pill, as a powder or as a dried herb extract. Dosing tends to be around 1 to 6grams per day.

Ashwagandha Tea

1.   Boil water.

2.   Add in 1 to 6grams per person of ashwagandha.

3.   Simmer for fifteen minutes.

4.   Strain and serve.

Ginkho Bilboa

Ginkgo Bilbao is an ancient herb which originates from China, and which has been used to treat a wide variety of health issues, for a period of thousands of years. Health conditions which are treatable include premenstrual tension, leg pain, vision problems, vertigo, dizziness and a movement disorder known as dyskinesia, to name but a few.

Ginkgo also appears to have a positive effect on a variety of mental health issues, which includes depression, anxiety and as a general stimulator of mental functioning. While there is a lack of scientific research verifying the potency of ginkgo, as a treatment for anxiety, there appears to be considerable anecdotal evidence to this effect.

How to use Ginkgo Bilbao:

Ginkgo comes in capsule form, powdered form and also as dried extract. For most people they will likely take capsules, although it is easy to make tea by supply boiling water, adding in a handful of dried leaves and leaving to simmer for fifteen minutes, prior to filtering and drinking.

Regarding dosing, doses for anxiety tend to be in the 80mg to 160mg up to three times per day.

Ginkgo Contraindications:

Major Interactions

• Ginkgo is potentially very dangerous when mixed with ibuprofen, as both ibuprofens and Ginkgo slows down clotting.

• Anticoagulant and antiplatelet medicine when combined with Ginkgo may result in excessive bleeding and bruising.

• Warfarin is used to slow blood clotting, so when combined with Ginkgo it could result in excessive bleeding and bursting.

Minor interactions

• Alprazolam (Xanax) Interacts badly with Ginkgo.

• Buspirone (BuSpar) Interacts badly with Ginkgo.

• Efavirenz (Sustiva) Interacts badly with Ginkgo.

- Fluoxetine (Prozac) Interacts badly with Ginkgo.

- Combining with St Johns wort may result in irritability in some cases.

- Some medications which are changed by the liver may interact badly with ginkgo.

Lemon Balm

Lemon balm is a perennial plant which belongs to the mint family. Lemon balm has many healing qualities which include enhancing skin vitality, liver boosting qualities and antioxidant properties. Lemon balm also contains a surprising number of mental health benefits which includes:

- Mind calming

- Treats insomnia

- Enhances alertness

- Improves memory

- Enhances problem solving abilities

Lemon balm (Melissa officinalis) is a powerful herb which has been clinically proven to have a good anti-depressive effect which is equivalent in potency to imipramine, which is a tricyclic dibenzazepine based anti-depressant. 16

How to Take Lemon Balm:

Lemon Balm can be taken in capsule form, tincture or it can be applied topically as a cream.

Lemon Balm Tea

1.   Boil water.

2.   Add in 1.5grams to 4.5grams of dried lemon balm into the water.

3.   Simmer for fifteen minutes.

4.   Strain and serve.

Capsules

Take 300 to 500mg three times daily.

Tinctures

1.   In order to make a tincture, it is necessary to mix the plant material with a liquid which will extract the compounds from the herb; this liquid is known as the menstrual. The ratio necessary with is 2:1. The menstruum can be alcohol; otherwise apple cider vinegar can be used instead. The menstruum also acts as a preserver, so the tincture can be used over a long period of time. Usually vodka, brandy or grain

alcohol are used as the alcohol base, do not use beer! It's necessary to have a fairly high percentage of alcohol, so as to preserve the tincture.

2.   To make up the menstruum, mix in alcohol/apple cider vinegar at the ratio of 3:1. So mix the alcohol and water at 3:1 and the menstruum with the lemon balm in a ratio of 2:1.

3.   Add in about 2 ounces (60grams) of lemon balm extract with 4 ounces of menstruum (about 3 ounces (90grams) of alcohol/vinegar to about 1 ounce (30 grams) of water. Place the mix into a blender and blend.

4.   Pour into a glass container (do not use plastic), leave in a dark cool place.

5.   Shake it daily for a period of 14 days.

6.   Strain through several layers of cheesecloth and squeeze out the essence.

7.   Leave this remaining mix to settle overnight, then pour out the clear liquid at the top (decant).

8.   Store in a dark glass container (a tincture bottle is ideal) in a cool dark place.

Dose: Lemon Balm
is usually taking as a tincture or as a tea. In tincture form, take 60 drops daily in a 2-4 millilitre tincture

Lemon Balm Contraindications:

- Lemon balm is basically safe, hoverer it can promote sleepiness and may result in over drowsiness if combined with sedatives.

Chapter Three – Final Considerations (How to Tackle Depression and Anxiety)

Hopefully you have found these herbal descriptions and recipes interesting send helpful.

So what next?

Take a look over chapter one again, as it is full of useful information and make a point of taking action, action is important, as it encourages empowerment.

Also you might feel daunted by the prospect of trying to make changes to your life there they be external life changes, such as where you work and live etc., and also internal life choices such as changing the way you think about yourself. Well this feeling of confusion and fear is quiet normal and to be expected.

What will help you to orientate yourself can be summed up in one word, which is:

RESPONSBILITY

The road to mental-emotional happiness lies in taking responsibility. In today's society it is all too easy to act like a victim and blame others for our problems. However, when we take responsibility, for our actions, then we actually empower ourselves.

Once again it's not the remit of this book to go into detail into this core value, which is an essential part of the self-healing process, but just think about it and try to apply it.

So for example, if your job sucks, rather than blaming your lousy boss on your troubles, just remind yourself that you chose to accept this job. If your marriage sucks, rather than blaming your problems upon your lousy spouse, remind yourself that you chose to accept them as a marriage partner, and if your unhappy where you live, rather than moaning about this lousy neighbourhood and the useless government, just take charge and move to another neighbourhood or make efforts to improve the neighbourhood or address the government by joining an action group, writing a letter to a major politician or government official etc.

The point is that depression and anxiety thrive on thoughts and feelings of self-disempowerment. Just start taking responsibility, for your actions, and you will be surprised at how much more empowered you can be and to what degree this will help with your life.

Now self-responsibility does not mean blame, we are not talking about blaming yourself and feeling bad, rather we are talking about taking responsibility for what you can do.

For example, you cannot make your boss fair minded, but you can be fair minded; you cannot make your spouse respect you, but you can chose whether or not you are going to respect them; you cannot control your neighbourhood but you can choose to either move neighbourhood or do something it improve your house, street etc.

So we are not supermen or superwomen, but we can take responsibility for whatever we can change in our life. It's not perfect but it is a good starting point.

If we look, for a minute, at the 12 steps as outlined by alcoholics anonymous (an organisation designed to help alcoholics heal themselves) we will note an emphasise upon self-responsibility.

1.   We admitted we were powerless over alcohol—that our lives had become unmanageable.

2.   Came to believe that a Power greater than ourselves could restore us to sanity.

3.   Made a decision to turn our will and our lives over to the care of God as we understood Him.

4.   Made a searching and fearless moral inventory of ourselves.

5.   Admitted to God, to ourselves, and to another human being the exact nature of our wrongs.

6.   Were entirely ready to have God remove all these defects of character.

7.   Humbly asked Him to remove our shortcomings.

8.   Made a list of all persons we had harmed, and became willing to make amends to them all.

9.   Made direct amends to such people wherever possible, except when to do so would injure them or others.

10.   Continued to take personal inventory, and when we were wrong, promptly admitted it.

11.   Sought through prayer and meditation to improve our conscious contact with God as we understood Him, praying only for knowledge of His will for us and the power to carry that out.

12.   Having had a spiritual awakening as the result of these steps, we tried to carry this message to alcoholics, and to practice these principles in all our affairs.

(The twelve steps are courtesy of www.aa.org)

Interestingly with a small change we can adjust the twelve steps so that it can help a person show is suffering from mental-emotional health issues, which is as follows:

1.   We admitted we were powerless over our mental health—that our lives had become unmanageable.

2.   Came to believe that a Power greater than ourselves could restore us to sanity.

3.   Made a decision to turn our will and our lives over to the care of God (or a higher power/higher self).

4.   Made a searching and fearless moral inventory of ourselves.

5.   Admitted to God (our higher power), to ourselves, and to another human being the exact nature of our wrongs.

6.   Were entirely ready to have God (our higher power), remove all these defects of character.

7.   Humbly asked Him to remove our shortcomings.

8.   Made a list of all persons we had harmed, and became willing to make amends to them all.

9.   Made direct amends to such people wherever possible, except when to do so would injure them or others.

10.   Continued to take personal inventory, and when we were wrong, promptly admitted it.

11.   Sought through prayer and meditation to improve our conscious contact with God (our higher power), as we understood Him, praying only for knowledge of His will for us and the power to carry that out.

12.   Having had a spiritual awakening, as the result of these steps, we tried to carry this message to other people with mental health issues, and to practice these principles in all our affairs.

Ok it might sound a little funny, in the way it is written, as the original 12 steps goes back to 1939, when people wrote this in an official manner and back when most people, in western society, where bible reading Sunday church going types. But don't let the datedness of the 12 steps fool you as they do actually work.

In the revised set of 12 steps I have added in higher power or higher self, in an effort to take the religious overtones out of the 12 steps. It's not so much about God, but rather about seeking some higher assistance and guidance which provides humility and much needed perspective, which is at the cornerstone of the 12 steps.

If we look at the 12 steps, in revised format, we see that the emphasize is on self-responsibility and on admitting that we have a problem and that it is outside of our conscious control to solve it. It's about sharing our problems with others and seeking help, it's about making reparation, it's about daily self-evaluation and it's about spreading the message of self-healing to others.

Its powerful stuff!

I first got introduced to the 12 step program back in 1994 when I was undergoing some counselling and although I have never had a problem with alcohol, I found the 12 steps to be a really easy and helpful way to start taking things in hand and re-empowering myself.

Also I picked up some nice thought for the day type books from both www.aa.org and also from http://www.hazelden.org/web/public/store.page . Reading these kinds of books can be a very helpful way of getting some perspective on our situation and in so doing so it can really help us to begin to see the wood for the treas.

Don't worry about the association of the 12 steps with alcohol and drug addiction. You might not be an alcoholic or a drug addict, but the same problems of disempowerment and escapism are prevalent. Mental health issue shares in common with alcohol and drug addiction a very strong mental element, whereby we have to adjust our thinking first and foremost, only then can we reshape our life.

The 12 steps might not be for you, I'm just putting it out there as a set of principles (which comes with a considerable amount of supporting literature) which may help you gain some traction over your mental-emotional wellbeing.

But even if you don't like the 12 steps, at least consider responsibility. Take responsibility, stop been a victim and start taking back control of your life.

The key feature of mental-emotional ill-health is a firm belief that we have no power and that we cannot do anything about it. Well yes you can do something about it, and you can start today!

Thank You

I hope you have enjoyed this book and found it interesting. These herbs are very powerful and are a simple way to support you through the recovery process. But do remember they are a support so don't simply swap allopathic medications for herbs. Both allopathic and herbal formulations are simply there to asset you while you recover.

If you like this book please leave a review for it and for more interesting and helpful information, on every suspect of physical, mental, emotional and spiritual health, please visit my website:

www.healbodymindandpspirit.com

Thanks once again for taking the time out to read this book.

Dermot Farrell

Free Gifts

Bonus #1 – Grab Free Books!!!!!!!!

As a way of saying thank you for downloading this book I would like to give you two free books, which are available exclusively for my readers. The free book "Juicing for Health – 35 Juicing Recipes for Everyday Health Problems", is packed full of useful healthy juice recipes and Success Hacks - 31 Mind-Set Hacks to Increase Productivity and Career Success, is packed full of helpful mind hacks for developing a more dynamic and enjoyable lifestyle!

Please go to my blog page and sign up here:

www.healbodymindandspirit.com

You will receive the two free eBooks, plus weekly updates and even free eBooks!

Bonus#2 - Bonus Video Series

You can check out my YouTube channel, which has lots of health related videos

Please copy the following link into your browser, to access an introduction to herbal remedies video. If you then go to my channel and click playlists, you will find lots of videos on herbs for health:

http://y2u.be/VJZ_Kc_dpL4

If you find it too awkward to type in this code, then you can also find my channel by typing in **www.healbodymindandspirit.com** into the YouTube search bar!

Dermot Farrell was born and raised in Ireland. He first took an interest in mental health back in the 1990's when he studied psychoanalytic studies, hypnotherapy and clinical psychoanalytical psychotherapy. While he learned a great deal about the workings of the mind, at this time, his interest in healing encouraged him to attend classes in Traditional Chinese Medicine and Acupuncture, finally culminating in him receiving a clinical diploma in 2005.

Since then Dermot has ran a TCM (Traditional Chinese Medical) clinic for a considerable period of time and also he has taken to writing about a variety of topics. His most recent writings are found on his blog www.healbodymindandspirit.com .

Dermot has learned, from his experience, the importance of balance in the three key domains of our life, which are physical, mental-emotional and spiritual wellbeing. His approach to healing is infinitely practical and is based upon the need to balance each of these aspects of our life, in order to regain a balanced state.

Furthermore, he is interested in moving the western/eastern medical discourse forward. Believing in the virtue of both western (allopathic) and eastern (complimentary) healing systems and is continually pushing for an integrated approach to healing. As the old saying goes "doctors differ, patients die!" demonstrates the need for everyone, who is interested in health and healing, to work together towards learning more about the causes of ill-health and the techniques of rebalancing health and reaching out in a humanistic way to help our patients, regain their health.

As well as his interest in healing Dermot possesses an interest in spirituality too. In 1999 Dermot began to meditate in an Indian system of Raja Yoga, known as Sahaj Marg. With an ardent interest in spirituality as well as physical, mental and emotional healing, Dermot presently resides in India with his wife and son.

Dermot can be contacted at admin@healbodymindandspirit.com

Website: www.healbodymindandspirit.com

Footnotes

Chapter Two – Anxiety

1.   Jerome Sarris, Con Stough, Chad A. Bousman, Zahra T. Wahid, Greg Murray, Rolf Teschke, Karen M. Savage, Ashley Dowell, Chee Ng, Isaac Schweitzer. Kava in the Treatment of Generalized Anxiety Disorder.Journal of Clinical Psychopharmacology, 2013; 1 DOI:

2.   Hyperforin, the active component of St. John's wort, induces IL-8 expression in human intestinal epithelial cells via a MAPK-dependent, NF-kappaB-independent pathway.

Zhou C1, Tabb MM, Sadatrafiei A, Grün F, Sun A, Blumberg B.

3.   Laakmann G, Schule C, Baghai T, et al. St. John's wort in mild to moderate depression: the relevance of hyperforin for the clinical efficacy. Pharmacopsychiat 1998; 31(suppl): 54-59.]

4.   Zaichikova SG, Grinkevich NI, Barabanov EI, et al. Healing properties and determination of the upper parameters of toxicity of Hypericum herb. Farmatsiya. 1985;34:62-64.

5.   Barbagallo C, Chisari G. Antimicrobial activity of three hypericum species.Fitoterapia. 1987;58:175-180.

6.   Razinkov SP, Yerofeyeva LN, Khovrina MP, Lazarev AI. Validation of the use of Hypericum perforatum medicamentous form with a prolonged action to treat patients with maxillary sinusitis. Zh Ushn Nos Gorl Bolezn. 1989;49:43-46.

7.   Martinez B, Kasper S, Ruhrmann S, Moller H-J. Hypericum in the treatment of seasonal affective disorders. Nervenheilkunde. 1993;12:302-307.

8.   Effect of valepotriates (valerian extract) in generalized anxiety disorder: a randomized placebo-controlled pilot study

Roberto Andreatini1,*, Vânia A. Sartori2,Maria L. V. Seabra2 andJosé Roberto Leite2

Article first published online: 30 OCT 2002

DOI: 10.1002/ptr.1027

9.   Pharmacopsychiatry. 2000 Mar;33(2):47-53.

Critical evaluation of the effect of valerian extract on sleep structure and sleep quality.

Donath F1, Quispe S, Diefenbach K, Maurer A, Fietze I, Roots I.

10.   Passionflower in the treatment of generalized anxiety: a pilot double-blind randomized controlled trial with oxazepam

S. Akhondzadeh PhD1,2, H. R. Naghavi MD1, M. Vazirian MD1, A. Shayeganpour PharmD2,

H. Rashidi PharmD2 andM. Khani MSc2

74

Article first published online: 12 JAN 2002

DOI: 10.1046/j.1365-2710.2001.00367.x

11.   Planta Med. 1995 Jun;61(3):213-6.

Apigenin, a component of Matricaria recutita flowers, is a central benzodiazepine receptors-ligand with anxiolytic effects.

Viola H1, Wasowski C, Levi de Stein M, Wolfman C, Silveira R, Dajas F, Medina JH, Paladini AC.

12.   Journal of Functional FoodsVolume 3, Issue 3, July 2011, Pages 171–178

Effects of L-theanine on attention and reaction time response

Akiko Higashiyamaa, Hla Hla Htayb, , , Makoto Ozekib, Lekh R. Junejab, Mahendra P. Kapoorb, ,

a University of Shiga Prefecture, Human Culture Department, Japan

b Taiyo Kagaku Co., Ltd., 1-3 Takaramachi, Yokkaichi, Mie 510-0844, Japan

Received 29 January 2010, Revised 22 February 2011, Accepted 23 March 2011, Available online 19 April 2011

13.   Effects of Aroma Inhalation Method on Test Anxiety, Stress Response and Serum Cortisol in Nursing Students

Journal title : Journal of Korean Academy of Fundamentals of Nursing

Volume 20, Issue 4, 2013, pp.410-418

75

Publisher : Korean Academy of Fundamentals of Nursing

DOI : 10.7739/jkafn.2013.20.4.410

Ko, Ye-Jung; Jung, Myoung-Soon; Park, Kyung-Sook;

14.   Antidepressant-like effects of an apolar extract and chow enriched with Nepeta cataria (catnip) in mice.

Bernardi, Maria Martha; Kirsten, Thiago Berti; Salzgeber, Simone Angélica;Ricci, Esther Lopes; Romoff, Paulete; Guilardi Lago, João Henrique; Lourenço, Lygia Mendes

Psychology & Neuroscience, Vol 3(2), Jul-Dec 2010, 251-258. http://dx.doi.org/10.3922/j.psns.2010.2.015

15.   Antistress, Adoptogenic and Immunopotentiating Activity Roots of Boerhaavia diffusa in Mice

Meera Sumanth, S.S. Mustafa

International Journal of Pharmacology

16.   DARU Journal of Pharmaceutical Sciences 2009. 17(1):42-47.

Antidepressant effect of Melissa officinalis in the forced swimming test

M Emamghoreishi , M.S Talebianpour